Gilbert's Syndrome: Causes, Tests and Treatment Options

Michael J. Harper, MA

Editor in Chief: *J.R. Hernandez, MD*

© 2012 Michael J. Harper

All Rights Reserved worldwide under the Berne Convention. May not be copied or distributed without prior written permission by the publisher. If you have this book or an electronic document and didn't pay for it, then the author didn't get a fair share. Please consider paying for your copy. Thank you!

Cover by euthman@flickr.com

Printed in the United States of America

ISBN 978-1470195311

Contents

Gilbert's Syndrome:

Learning the Basics and Taking Precautions for Healthy Living

The liver is one of the busiest and most important organs in your body. When it functions properly, it detoxifies harmful substances and filters impurities, stores energy, processes carbohydrates, and breaks down fats. To help you digest your food, a yellowish brown fluid in the gallbladder is discharged to break down fats and lipids in the intestines. Unfortunately, a common, mild disorder may take place causing this yellowish-brown pigment in the bile to increase in high levels. This pigment—known as bilirubin—causes the skin and whites of the eyes to turn yellow or jaundiced. A person with this kind of disorder is thought to have an inherited Gilbert's syndrome (GS).

In many cases, Gilbert's syndrome is so mild thus giving no obvious symptoms. Most of the cases are diagnosed by accident when blood tests are undertaken to investigate for unrelated illnesses. Despite the person's jaundiced appearance, the liver still functions normally. Though Gilbert's syndrome is considered harmless, it is imperative to acquire appropriate information regarding this syndrome. Proper awareness and thorough knowledge on this disorder will help you receive proper medication and avoid complications.

Here are important points that you need to know regarding Gilbert's syndrome. These will help you lead a healthy life and uphold wellness for better living.

Overview and Causes of GS

Augustine Nicolas Gilbert, a French gastroenterologist and his colleagues, first described Gilbert's syndrome (GS) in 1901. The disorder was first recognized as a syndrome of chronic, benign, intermittent yellowing of the skin and whites of the eyes or jaundice in the absence of other liver diseases. In addition, they also described psychological symptoms including signs of chronic fatigue syndrome which refers to painful muscles and nerve inflammation.

a. Background on bilirubin

Gilbert's syndrome starts with an increased level of bilirubin in the bloodstreams. To fully understand this disorder, it would be very helpful to trace the means on how this pigment increases in level.

Bilirubin is considered a normal by-product of iron breakdown in the blood. It is created in the natural breakdown of red blood cells (RBCs) in the spleen. These cells contain hemoglobin which is an important protein that helps transport oxygen all over the body. After 120 days, the red blood cells break into *globin*, a protein, and *haem*, a waste material. To undergo further chemical changes, *haem* is transported to the liver and becomes the bilirubin in the bile while the protein is stored in the liver for future use. This will be excreted from the body.

Together with other toxins and impurities, bilirubin is treated in the body's two-phase detoxification system. The body may detoxify toxins entirely in the first phase or prepare it for the second phase. Several major systems act on these toxins in the second phase. If you are affected with Gilbert's syndrome, the system that is responsible for processing toxins and removing them in the body is not functioning well. This is known to take place in the *glucuronidation* system and enzymes in this system are called *uridine diphosphate glucuronyl transferase* or UGT. A specific enzyme in this family is responsible in breaking down and modifying bilirubin into a water-soluble form. Bilirubin in watery version is secreted easily into bile through your gall bladder and into your small intestine. It is further acted by bacteria into forms of pigment substances and eventually excreted from the body in your feces and urine.

In Gilbert's syndrome, a genetic mutation takes place that triggers only 30% of the UGT enzyme to be produced and act on the toxins. There are not enough UGT enzymes to metabolize bilirubin at the normal rate. The shortage in this type of enzyme leads to an excess of bilirubin in the blood serum. With this disorder, your liver has problems with chemical conversion and abnormally high amounts of bilirubin will circulate in the bloodstream. This causes yellowing of the skin and the whites of the eyes. In some cases, the bilirubin levels typically fluctuate and only sometimes drift within the normal range.

b. Risk factors: how is GS is passed through families?

Although studies link genetic mutation with the causes of Gilbert's syndrome, further researches are conducted to explain thoroughly the exact causes of this disorder. At present, most experts and researchers point out that poor enzyme function has family history in most cases. In this case, Gilbert's syndrome is considered to be an inherited disorder.

Experts say that GS is a finding, not a disease. This is found in about five percent of the population. While both sexes are affected by GS, it takes place twenty five percent more in men than in women. They tend to develop this disorder between late teens and early thirties.

The gene that carries and causes GS is common. This abnormal gene is present in more than fifty percent of the population. To inherit Gilbert's syndrome, two copies of these abnormal genes are required. Therefore, if two individuals are carriers and they produce a child, they may pass the genetic defect that triggers Gilbert's syndrome to their offspring. Nonetheless, this is not true in all cases and not everyone who carries two copies develops the disorder. So, there is a possibility that an individual may acquire such condition without a family history of it.

Signs and Symptoms of GS

In most cases, Gilbert's syndrome is so mild and typically causes no obvious signs and symptoms. Opinions on the symptoms associated with GS vary among experts. If GS causes the level of bilirubin in the bloodstreams increase enough, you may experience jaundice or a yellowish tinged in your skin and whites of your eyes. Some observed that yellowing of the whites of the eyes is more dominant than on the skin. Other possible symptoms may include abdominal pain, anxiety, fatigue, nausea and weakness.

Aside from these typical symptoms, you should take into consideration some factors that may contribute to increase in symptoms. These are alcohol intake, dehydration, fasting, illnesses including infections such as cold or flu, overexertion and menstruation.

Survey on GS' symptoms

To study further on the symptoms of Gilbert's syndrome, a survey was conducted of 286 people with the disorder. This survey is a limited one and the list of symptoms is not exhaustive. Despite the limits, this survey can provide concrete evidence on the degree of GS and identify common signs across the population. The following symptoms will help you identify signs that in one way or the other can be attributed to GS.

a. Frequently reported symptoms

1. Fatigue, tiredness and jaundice
2. Brain fog and poor memory
3. Headache, dizziness or nausea
4. Irritability, depression, anxiety, tremors and itchiness
5. Loss of appetite, irritable bowel syndrome and abdominal pain
6. Stomach cramping, liver/ gallbladder pain

b. Commonly reported symptoms

1. Insomnia, panic attacks, difficulty concentrating

2. Hypoglycemic reaction to foods, carbohydrates and alcohol intolerance

3. Loose stools or diarrhea, abdominal bloating or swelling

4. Heart palpitations, breathlessness or labored breathing

5. Aching muscles, body aches and joint pain

6. Weakness, numbness or tingling sensation

7. Chemical sensitivity, weight loss, feeling constantly sick

c. Sometimes reported symptoms

1. Difficulty finding the right words, feeling drunk, strong hangovers

2. Acid reflux, excessive thirst, chest pain

3. Muscle twitches, cold hands and feet

4. Environmental allergies, swollen lymph nodes

5. Toxic feeling or metallic taste in the mouth, eye pain

d. Occasionally reported symptoms

1. Mood swings, feeling antisocial, waking panic attack
2. Intolerance to drugs, constipation, pale stools and indigestion
3. Dry skin, low body temperature and pale skin
4. Low weight, night sweats, sore or dry throat
5. Light sensitivity, poor immune system, bloodshot eyes

The aforementioned signs and symptoms are grouped and analyzed to determine their causes. Sensitivity and intolerance are linked to reduced liver function while appetite and weight issues are linked to gastroparesis. Most of the sub-effects are known to be caused by heartburn and acid reflux disease. Abnormal bowel movements are associated with digestive problems without a known cause. Since doctors consider GS to be asymptomatic; more studies are conducted to explain these symptoms and draw a clearer link to the syndrome.

Diagnosis and Tests

Most cases of Gilbert's syndrome are discovered by chance when blood testing is conducted for unrelated diseases such as in Complete Blood Count (CBC). Some are also discovered if high levels of bilirubin are detected in the blood during liver function test. Generally, these tests give out normal results except for a slightly elevated content of unconjugated bilirubin (UCB). In addition, this syndrome can be diagnosed by a thorough history and physical examinations. There are no invasive procedures that are justified for establishing diagnosis of Gilbert's syndrome.

Gilbert's syndrome is usually detected around puberty. This is possible because of various hormonal changes during this period and inhibition of bilirubin metabolisms by endogenous steroid hormones. The disorder is usually diagnosed in adults in line with routine blood test results or discovered by inter-current illness or stress. GS occurs predominantly in men gaining a male-to-female ratio ranging from 2:1 or 7:1. Furthermore, GS is not restricted to any ethnic group and can occur in all races and in any person.

To get better diagnosis of GS, it is best to be tested for liver and blood problems and bilirubin levels. The liver test is known as a "liver function testing". For a bilirubin test, your blood is examined for its total, conjugated and unconjugated levels. In other cases, GS may be accompanied by similar to more serious liver diseases, so appropriate medical attention must be provided. Common diagnostic tests may include medical history evaluation, physical and blood examination and urinalysis. A clinician may also order ultrasound of the liver and bile ducts to make sure there are no other causes of high levels of bilirubin. Although a genetic test can be used to detect the abnormal gene that causes GS, it is usually unnecessary for diagnosis and is not widely available.

While GS is not considered a serious disorder, it is still important to manage the symptom and take control over the syndrome. When experiencing jaundice, it is important to know the following conditions that can cause the yellowing of your skin and whites of the eyes in order to distinguish them from Gilbert's syndrome.

a. **Hepatitis.** An inflammation of the liver cells specifically caused by viral infection of hepatitis A, B, C, or others. This damage of the liver can also be drug-induced, for example paracetamol poisoning. These factors damage the liver cells causing inability to process bilirubin to into its simpler form.

b. **Blockage of the bile flow (cholestasis).** A system of ducts serves as passage of bile as it leaves the liver. This pathway is initially composed of very tiny ducts that make up a linkage and eventually form the main bile duct. This duct connects to the digestive system just beyond the outlet of the stomach. Blockage of the bile duct will hinder the processing of bile into useful forms and contribute to the increased levels of bilirubin in the bloodstreams. The blockage can occur for several reasons including gallstones.

c. **Excessive breakdown of red blood cells (hemolysis).** The regular red cell life of 120 days may be shortened due to some drugs or in a condition called hemolytic anemia. Nonetheless, drug-induced causes are rare side effects.

Treatment for Gilbert's Syndrome

Gilbert's Syndrome is a mild disorder and normally does not need medical treatment. Most of patients with the disorder continue to live normal, healthy lives. So far, there is no evidence to suggest that the condition is harmful or may lead to more serious disease. Nonetheless, there might be very rare cases of complications and consequences. Medications can be employed to help lower bilirubin levels. There are also drugs that may aid to reduce jaundice if this becomes a problem. The bilirubin content in your blood may fluctuate over time and you may only occasionally experience jaundice. The yellowing of the skin and whites of the eyes usually goes away on its own and doesn't require treatment.

Management of Gilbert's Syndrome

In order to take over symptoms and control GS, your doctor may require you to change lifestyle and observe dos and don'ts. The following diet supplements will help you control symptoms and manage this disorder.

a. *What could make you feel worse?*

1. **Alcohol.** When acquiring GS, you seem sensitive to alcohol to differing degrees. Therefore, you should be aware that alcohol can cause and add stress to your liver.

2. **Fatty Foods.** For GS cases, digestive problems are common and you may find fatty foods putting more pressure on your digestive system. So, to aid in the digestion of your food, avoid fatty foods.

3. **Sweetened or sugary foods and refined carbohydrates.** These foods mess with your energy levels and if you're suffering from fatigue, eating these foods will not help you balance your energy. In addition, sugar can impair the ability of your liver to detoxify toxins and impurities.

4. **Artificial sweeteners** can cause increase the occurrence of the 'brain-fog' experience. On the other hand, taking the B vitamin niacin on its own can be detrimental to your liver but it would be acceptable if taken with other B vitamins. Other materials that should be avoided are fluoride, peppermint, vanilla and menthol.

b. ***What could help you?***

1. Increasing the proportion of your protein diet may raise energy levels. It is noted that oily fish may be particularly effective as it could also enhance the removal of the fat-soluble from the body.

2. Maintain a healthy diet that is good for your liver. This often includes legumes, whole grains, lecithin, fruits and vegetables. You are advised to maintain a diet rich in raw fruits and vegetables with emphasis on green leafy vegetables. These are powerful healing tools and increase elimination of toxins and waste products from skin while improving the function of liver, bowels and kidneys.

3. Drink eight glasses of water every day. Purified water with lemon is also excellent for you. Avoid all processed foods such as refined sugar, fried food, junk food, coffee tea and soft drinks. Eating small regular meals is recommended rather than over-eating.

4. Aim to limit dairy products since they contain high levels of steroids, artificial growth hormones and antibiotics. This is the result of treatment that herds receive to prevent disease and boost milk production.

5. You should avoid all margarines and similar spreads of the same type manufactured from hydrogenated fats.

6. Avoid deep fried and fatty foods. Also, limit intake food from chicken, turkey and eggs that are not organic because these contain steroids and artificial growth hormones. These may increase the liver's workload.

7. Taurine plays a major factor in good liver function through detoxification while turmeric has been shown to increase glutathione and other enzymes important for detoxification. Glutathione (GSH) is known to be the most powerful internal antioxidant and liver protector.

8. A combination of those containing glutathione and natural sulfur compounds will help in the breakdown of chemicals and impurities. Examples are broccoli, avocadoes, cabbage, walnuts, eggs, blueberries and cauliflower.

9. To enhance detoxification in the phase 2 pathways, production of glutathione must be increased. This can be acquired in supplements of glutamic acid, cysteine and glycine.

10. You can also use milk thistle as herbal remedy for liver disorders and depression. Most medicinal herbalists recommend this medication for depression.

11. Carrots and beetroot are good detox aids.

12. Methionine, an amino acid, also activates the phase 2 pathways for thorough oxidation.

13. Dandelion tea can stimulate liver function.

14. You can also find energy benefits in taking Royal Jelly.

In dealing with GS symptoms, you should lead a healthy lifestyle. The following ideas will help you maintain a well-balanced life while having Gilbert's syndrome.

a. Exercise will serve you better when you do it gradually. You can benefit more when you gently increase your fitness level over time. Avoid sudden exertion because this will surely cause fatigue. In doing exercise every day, you will observe that there is an increase in your energy level and improvement in your ability to exert oneself more than previously, without the same consequences. Doing good exercise for at least 30 minutes a day is advised.

b. Have enough sleep as much as you can. If you are experiencing symptoms, you need to sleep at least 8 hours a day so you can regain energy. When you lack sleep, your liver functions are stressed. This will eventually result to GS symptoms over time. If you are used to struggling at the end of the day, taking a nap after lunch would be helpful in preserving energy levels for the evening.

c. Overcome anxiety, stress and depression. After you experience GS symptoms, you may suffer socio-phobia and anxiety attacks. This will lead to psychological stress and raise mental health issues. Both will result to unhappiness that creates physical responses leading to stressing the liver function and trigger symptoms.

d. Get a balance with work, rest and play.

Studies discovered that despite its sometimes uncomfortable symptoms, GS is not that dangerous. Some experts even say that normally, this disorder won't harm your liver, make you sick or shorten your life. It is an important precaution that you make sure your physician know that you have Gilbert's syndrome. In this way, your doctor can prescribe medications that will not worsen the disorder since the enzyme responsible also acts on the medications that your body is taking. If your doctor is not aware of your condition, he may order other clinical tests that are not necessary.

Moreover, no herbs or supplements are needed to address your condition although the aforementioned supplements and herbs (like milk thistle) may help. You can prevent the increase of bilirubin content in your body by avoiding flu and colds, staying hydrated with purified drinking water, keeping a balanced diet and avoiding strenuous activity. Since there is no specific treatment for Gilbert's syndrome, you can still effectively handle the disorder by managing symptoms. Seek help from your doctor to help you manage anxiety, stress and depression. Many organizations are giving better advice and you can also join groups in meditation, yoga, cognitive behavioral therapy and other forms of dealing with your frame of mind.

Complications and relations to other disorders

Gilbert's syndrome can cause fluctuations of jaundice. You may experience episodes of yellowing of the skin and whites of the eyes but this is usually mild and goes away on its own. For extremely elevated bilirubin levels, your doctor may prescribe phenobarbital to reduce signs of jaundice.

a. Side effects with certain medications

Since GS symptoms are caused by low levels of bilirubin-processing enzymes, this can cause increased side effects with certain medications. These effects are triggered because the certain enzymes also play a major role in eliminating these medications from your body. Certain drugs that are broken down by the liver can increase risk of side effects.

Cancer chemotherapy drugs such as Camptosar or irinotecan can enhance and reach toxic levels if you have Gilbert's syndrome. This treatment may cause severe diarrhea. Medications used in HIV patients such as Crixivan or indinavir can also cause complications in patients who have Gilbert's syndrome.

With potential side effects of certain medications, you should talk to your doctor and check with your healthcare provider before taking any medications.

b. Known effects of Gilbert's Syndrome

The following describe observed effects of GS through a survey given to people with the syndrome. Awareness on these effects may help you assess your condition and take appropriate actions together with your doctor in order to avoid these possible effects.

1. **Swollen Liver or Liver Hypertrophy.** This condition occurs due to increase in cell size of the liver rather than division. With ultrasonographic examinations, results reveal that there is a significantly larger anteroposterior dimension of the right liver lobe by 11%. This right lobe is observed to be larger than the other side. This increased size of the organ should be distinguished from hyperplasia which occurs due to cell division.

2. **Liver Webs.** With electron microscopy (EM), it is observed that formation of liver webs disturb bile flow. This will hinder the liver to release bile therefore increasing bilirubin levels that are not processed further.

3. Increased toxicity of certain medications. Recent studies suggest that you may show increased toxicity compared to unaffected individuals. This is triggered by use of medications which are metabolized by the liver. This is related with anti-cancer agents and paracetamol. You are exposed to toxicity after a paracetamol overdose.

4. Severe Jaundice. The yellowing of the skin can cause a feeling of itchiness and can be linked to dark urine and light stools. Aside from the cosmetic issues of looking yellow, the itching associated with jaundice can sometimes be severe. This can cause you scratching your skin raw and you can have trouble in sleeping.

5. Increased neonatal jaundice. Although jaundice levels do not differ among races of individuals, newborn infants with positive marker of GS may appear yellow. This catalyzes in the increased neonatal jaundice during the first two days of life.

6. Essential Tremors. With higher baseline level of bilirubin, you may experience distinct response to functional test and medication acted by the enzyme responsible. This is frequently combined with essential tremors.

7. Immune Suppression. A study conducted provides basis that the bilirubin infusion both in the inductive and productive phase decreased significantly the immune responses. It can be assumed that bilirubin influences the differentiation of competent cells in the immune system immediately after contact with antigen.

8. Increased hemolysis. Moderately shortened erythrocyte life span has been discovered during a study. This happened to 61% of the patients that increase bile pigment production. Nevertheless, biochemical assays revealed that there might be disturbed bilirubin metabolisms but other functions of the liver cells are normal

9. Gastroparesis or delayed gastric emptying. Increase in bilirubin in the body can decrease intestinal motility. Studies revealed that as a GS sufferer, you have the tendency to have a shorter intestinal transit time so the stomach takes longer to empty whatever meal has been eaten. This explains why you feel full easily and you tend to eat little. In addition, this also implies that if you eat a large meal, you may suffer from heartburn since the stomach is full longer.

10. Increased risk of gallstones. The defect in the waste removal of the liver has a possible role in initiating buildup of cholesterol gallstones. According to studies conducted, 25% of those with gallstones had GS, while only 3% of those are negative for the syndrome. Moreover, 15% of the stones are composed of bilirubin and most of the cholesterol stones in the gallbladder found to have bilirubin center. This proves that the gallstones are triggered by increased bilirubin contents and this can lead to gallstone initiation regardless of the composition of the stone.

c. **Relations to other disorders**

1. Leaky Gut Syndrome. In some cases, the taxing of the liver is linked to GS. This is related to symptoms of food allergies, stomach discomfort, acid reflux disease and delayed gastric emptying.

2. Adrenal Fatigue. After symptoms attack, there can be extreme adrenal exhaustion with increased blood pressure. With GS, there is fluctuation of anxiety levels, heart palpitations and other physical and emotional reactions caused by action of enzymes responsible in the disorder.

3. Fibroids. Recent evidence linked GS with enlargement of fibroids (non cancerous growths in the uterus). A case on this condition has been reported that needed to have a hysterectomy (surgical removal of the uterus). This is sometimes caused by treatments that put too much pressure on the body organs such as bowels, livers, bladder and the kidneys. Condition in GS can greatly affect detoxification of estrogen. The excess in estrogen is considered to cause growth in fibroids.

4. **Seasonal Affective disorder (SAD).** A study revealed that patients with SAD are actually displaying lower nighttime bilirubin levels. Similarly, SAD patients who are exposed to a light source which is a common treatment for the disorder have been observed to demonstrate increased levels of bilirubin. Excess bilirubin triggers seasonal depression. More females are affected with SAD and are observed to be afflicted by this disorder during winter lacking energy and interest in work.

Yoga

Yoga is a mind-body practice in complementary and alternative medicine (CAM) with origins in ancient Indian philosophy. The various styles of yoga that people use for health purposes typically combine physical postures, breathing techniques, and meditation or relaxation. There are numerous schools of yoga. Hatha yoga, the most commonly practiced in the United States and Europe, emphasizes postures (*asanas*) and breathing exercises (*pranayama*). Some of the major styles of hatha yoga include Iyengar, Ashtanga, Vini, Kundalini, and Bikram yoga. People use yoga for a variety of conditions and to achieve fitness and relaxation.

The 2007 National Health Interview Survey found that yoga is one of the top 10 CAM modalities used among U.S. adults. An estimated 6 percent of adults used yoga for health purposes in the previous 12 months.

- People use yoga for a variety of health conditions and to achieve fitness and relaxation.

- It is not fully known what changes occur in the body during yoga; whether they influence health; and if so, how. There is, however, growing evidence to suggest that yoga works to enhance stress-coping mechanisms and mind-body awareness. Research is under way to find out more about yoga's effects, and the diseases and conditions for which it may be most helpful.

- Tell your health care providers about any complementary and alternative practices you use. Give them a full picture of what you do to manage your health. This will help ensure coordinated and safe care.

Overview

Yoga in its full form combines physical postures, breathing exercises, meditation, and a distinct philosophy. Yoga is intended to increase relaxation and balance the mind, body, and the spirit.

Early written descriptions of yoga are in Sanskrit, the classical language of India. The word "yoga" comes from the Sanskrit word *yuj*, which means "yoke or union." It is believed that this describes the union between the mind and the body. The first known text, *The Yoga Sutras*, was written more than 2,000 years ago, although yoga may have been practiced as early as 5,000 years ago. Yoga was originally developed as a method of discipline and attitudes to help people reach spiritual enlightenment. The *Sutras* outline eight limbs or foundations of yoga practice that serve as spiritual guidelines:

1. *yama* (moral behavior)
2. *niyama* (healthy habits)
3. *asana* (physical postures)
4. *pranayama* (breathing exercises)
5. *pratyahara* (sense withdrawal)
6. *dharana* (concentration)
7. *dhyana* (contemplation)
8. *samadhi* (higher consciousness)

The numerous schools of yoga incorporate these eight limbs in varying proportions. Hatha yoga, the most commonly practiced in the United States and Europe, emphasizes two of the eight limbs: postures (*asanas*) and breathing exercises (*pranayama*). Some of the major styles of hatha yoga include Ananda, Anusara, Ashtanga, Bikram, Iyengar, Kripalu, Kundalini, and Viniyoga.

Use of Yoga for Health in the United States

According to the 2007 National Health Interview Survey (NHIS), which included a comprehensive survey of CAM use by Americans, yoga is one of the top 10 CAM modalities used. More than 13 million adults had used yoga in the previous year, and between the 2002 and 2007 NHIS, use of yoga among adults increased by 1 percent (or approximately 3 million people). The 2007 survey also found that more than 1.5 million children used yoga in the previous year.

People use yoga for a variety of health conditions including anxiety disorders or stress, asthma, high blood pressure, and depression. People also use yoga as part of a general health regimen—to achieve physical fitness and to relax.

The Status of Yoga Research

Research suggests that yoga might:

- Improve mood and sense of well-being
- Counteract stress
- Reduce heart rate and blood pressure
- Increase lung capacity
- Improve muscle relaxation and body composition
- Help with conditions such as anxiety, depression, and insomnia
- Improve overall physical fitness, strength, and flexibility
- Positively affect levels of certain brain or blood chemicals.

More well-designed studies are needed before definitive conclusions can be drawn about yoga's use for specific health conditions.

Side Effects and Risks

Yoga is generally considered to be safe in healthy people

when practiced appropriately. Studies have found it to be well tolerated, with few side effects.

- People with certain medical conditions should not use some yoga practices. For example, people with disc disease of the spine, extremely high or low blood pressure, glaucoma, retinal detachment, fragile or atherosclerotic arteries, a risk of blood clots, ear problems, severe osteoporosis, or cervical spondylitis should avoid some inverted poses.

- Although yoga during pregnancy is safe if practiced under expert guidance, pregnant women should avoid certain poses that may be problematic.

Training, Licensing, and Certification

There are many training programs for yoga teachers throughout the country. These programs range from a few days to more than 2 years. Standards for teacher training and certification differ depending on the style of yoga.

There are organizations that register yoga teachers and training programs that have complied with minimum educational standards. For example, one nonprofit group requires at least 200 hours of training, with a specified number of hours in areas including techniques, teaching methodology, anatomy, physiology, and philosophy. However, there are currently no official or well-accepted licensing requirements for yoga teachers in the United States.

If You Are Thinking About Yoga

- Do not use yoga as a replacement for conventional care or to postpone seeing a doctor about a medical problem.
- If you have a medical condition, consult with your health care provider before starting yoga.
- Ask about the physical demands of the type of yoga in which you are interested, as well as the training and experience of the yoga teacher you are considering.
- Look for published research studies on yoga for the health condition you are interested in.
- Tell your health care providers about any complementary and alternative practices you use. Give them a full picture of what you do to manage your health. This will help ensure coordinated and safe care.

NCCAM-Funded Research

Recent studies supported by NCCAM have been investigating yoga's effects on:

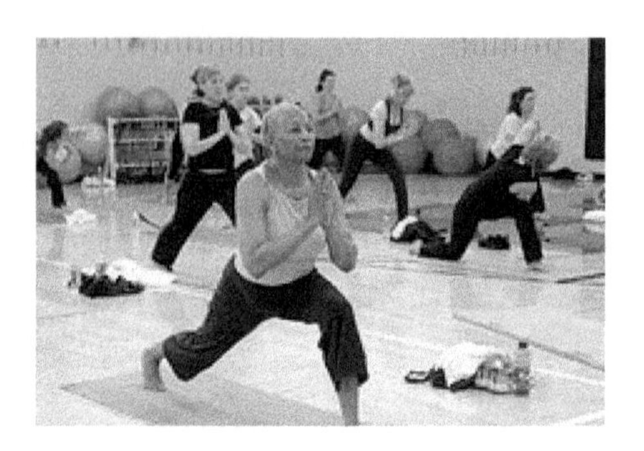

Women in yoga class

Courtesy of National Institute on Aging

- Blood pressure
- Chronic low-back pain
- Chronic obstructive pulmonary disease
- Depression
- Diabetes risk
- HIV
- Immune function
- Inflammatory arthritis and knee osteoarthritis
- Insomnia

- Multiple sclerosis
- Smoking cessation.

Meditation

Meditation is known to be a very powerful tool to counter pain with. At first, it certainly will seem very hard but with practice, if can become a powerful tool to combat pain. Meditation is a mind-body practice in complementary and alternative medicine (CAM). There are many types of meditation, most of which originated in ancient religious and spiritual traditions. Generally, a person who is meditating uses certain techniques, such as a specific posture, focused attention, and an open attitude toward distractions. Meditation may be practiced for many reasons, such as to increase calmness and physical relaxation, to improve psychological balance, to cope with illness, or to enhance overall health and well-being. This Backgrounder provides a general introduction to meditation and suggests some resources for more information.

- People practice meditation for a number of health-related purposes.

- It is not fully known what changes occur in the body during meditation; whether they influence health; and, if so, how. Research is under way to find out more about meditation's effects, how it works, and diseases and conditions for which it may be most helpful.

- Tell your health care providers about any complementary and alternative practices you use. Give them a full picture of what you do to manage your health. This will help ensure coordinated and safe care.

The term *meditation* refers to a group of techniques, such as mantra meditation, relaxation response, mindfulness meditation, and Zen Buddhist meditation. Most meditative techniques started in Eastern religious or spiritual traditions. These techniques have been used by many different cultures throughout the world for thousands of years. Today, many people use meditation outside of its traditional religious or cultural settings, for health and well-being.

In meditation, a person learns to focus attention. Some forms of meditation instruct the practitioner to become mindful of thoughts, feelings, and sensations and to observe them in a nonjudgmental way. This practice is believed to result in a state of greater calmness and physical relaxation, and psychological balance. Practicing meditation can change how a person relates to the flow of emotions and thoughts.

Most types of meditation have four elements in common:

- **A quiet location.** Meditation is usually practiced in a quiet place with as few distractions as possible. This can be particularly helpful for beginners.
- **A specific, comfortable posture.** Depending on the type being practiced, meditation can be done while sitting, lying down, standing, walking, or in other positions.
- **A focus of attention.** Focusing one's attention is usually a part of meditation. For example, the meditator may focus on a mantra (a specially chosen word or set of words), an object, or the sensations of the breath. Some forms of meditation involve paying attention to whatever is the dominant content of consciousness.
- **An open attitude.** Having an open attitude during meditation means letting distractions come and go naturally without judging them. When the attention goes to distracting or wandering thoughts, they are not suppressed; instead, the meditator gently brings attention back to the focus. In some types of meditation, the meditator learns to "observe" thoughts and emotions while meditating.

Meditation used as CAM is a type of mind-body medicine. Generally, mind-body medicine focuses on:

- The interactions among the brain/mind, the rest of the body, and behavior.
- The ways in which emotional, mental, social, spiritual, and behavioral factors can directly affect health.

Uses of Meditation for Health in the United States

A 2007 national Government survey that asked about CAM use in a sample of 23,393 U.S. adults found that 9.4 percent of respondents (representing more than 20 million people) had used meditation in the past 12 months—compared with 7.6 percent of respondents (representing more than 15 million people) in a similar survey conducted in 2002. The 2007 survey also asked about CAM use in a sample of 9,417 children; 1 percent (representing 725,000 children) had used meditation in the past 12 months.

People use meditation for various health problems, such as:

- Anxiety
- Pain

- Depression
- Stress
- Insomnia
- Physical or emotional symptoms that may be associated with chronic illnesses (such as heart disease, HIV/AIDS, and cancer) and their treatment.

Meditation is also used for overall wellness.

Examples of Meditation Practices

Mindfulness meditation and Transcendental Meditation (also known as TM) are two common forms of meditation. NCCAM-sponsored research projects are studying both types of meditation.

Mindfulness meditation is an essential component of Buddhism. In one common form of mindfulness meditation, the meditator is taught to bring attention to the sensation of the flow of the breath in and out of the body. The meditator learns to focus attention on what is being experienced, without reacting to or judging it. This is seen as helping the meditator learn to experience thoughts and emotions in normal daily life with greater balance and acceptance.

The TM technique is derived from Hindu traditions. It uses a mantra (a word, sound, or phrase repeated silently) to prevent distracting thoughts from entering the mind. The goal of TM is to achieve a state of relaxed awareness.

How Meditation Might Work

Practicing meditation has been shown to induce some changes in the body. By learning more about what goes on in the body during meditation, researchers hope to be able to identify diseases or conditions for which meditation might be useful.

Some types of meditation might work by affecting the autonomic (involuntary) nervous system. This system regulates many organs and muscles, controlling functions such as heartbeat, sweating, breathing, and digestion. It has two major parts:

- The **sympathetic nervous system** helps mobilize the body for action. When a person is under stress, it produces the "fight-or-flight response": the heart rate and breathing rate go up and blood vessels narrow (restricting the flow of blood).
- The **parasympathetic nervous system** causes the heart rate and breathing rate to slow

down, the blood vessels to dilate (improving blood flow), and the flow of digestive juices increases.

It is thought that some types of meditation might work by reducing activity in the sympathetic nervous system and increasing activity in the parasympathetic nervous system.

In one area of research, scientists are using sophisticated tools to determine whether meditation is associated with significant changes in brain function. A number of researchers believe that these changes account for many of meditation's effects.

It is also possible that practicing meditation may work by improving the mind's ability to pay attention. Since attention is involved in performing everyday tasks and regulating mood, meditation might lead to other benefits.

A 2007 NCCAM-funded review of the scientific literature found some evidence suggesting that meditation is associated with potentially beneficial health effects. However, the overall evidence was inconclusive. The reviewers concluded that future research needs to be more rigorous before firm conclusions can be drawn.

Side Effects and Risks

Meditation is considered to be safe for healthy people. There have been rare reports that meditation could cause or worsen symptoms in people who have certain psychiatric problems, but this question has not been fully researched. People with physical limitations may not be able to participate in certain meditative practices involving physical movement. Individuals with existing mental or physical health conditions should speak with their health care providers prior to starting a meditative practice and make their meditation instructor aware of their condition.

If You Are Thinking About Using Meditation Practices

- Do not use meditation as a replacement for conventional care or as a reason to postpone seeing a doctor about a medical problem.

- Ask about the training and experience of the meditation instructor you are considering.

- Look for published research studies on meditation for the health condition in which you are interested.

- Tell all your health care providers about any complementary and alternative practices you use. Give them a full picture of what you do to manage your health. This will help ensure coordinated and safe care. For tips about talking with your health care providers about CAM, see NCCAM's Time to Talk campaign at http://nccam.nih.gov/timetotalk/.

NCCAM-Supported Research

Some recent NCCAM-supported studies have been investigating meditation for:

- Relieving stress in caregivers for elderly patients with dementia
- Reducing the frequency and intensity of hot flashes in menopausal women
- Relieving symptoms of chronic back pain
- Improving attention-related abilities (alerting, focusing, and prioritizing)
- Relieving asthma symptoms.

Prognosis and Prevalence of Gilbert's syndrome

According to studies and researches, this genetic disorder is common and benign. The condition of the processing enzymes and bilirubin disposition may be regarded as falling within the range of normal biologic fluctuation or variations. The syndrome is known to generally not be serious or life threatening. There is an excellent outlook for GS patients and you likely can lead a normal lifestyle. Successful liver transplants from donors with Gilbert's syndrome have confirmed the benign nature of GS.

Prevalence of Gilbert's syndrome in the United States is three to seven percent. Globally, the prevalence varies considerably depending on diagnostic criteria used. Common criteria used include levels of bilirubin determinations, method of analysis, fasting of the patient and bilirubin levels used for diagnosis. Thirty six percent of African and three percent of Asians are affected by a portion of the abnormal gene that promotes further complications of the disorder. Molecular genetics studies are conducted to explain this promoter region caused by polymorphisms. Moreover, clinical phenotype may not be that useful in determining genotype because of the other factors. This includes environmental influences such as alcohol-induced bilirubin that can reduce bilirubin levels.

Recipe Suggestions

Breakfast

Mango Smoothie

2 cups yogurt
2 cups chopped fresh mango
1 Tbsp flax seeds 1/2 cup ice
1 Tbsp agave nectar

Procedure

1 Combine all ingredients in a blender and blend until smooth and flax seeds are ground.

Servings: 4
Yield: 4
Preparation Time: 5 minutes

Nutrition Facts

Serving size: 1/4 of a recipe (7.8 ounces).
Calories:186.08
Calories from fat:35.41
Carbs:34.51g
Protein: 5.48g

Spinach Frittata

1/3 cup vegetable broth
2 medium potatoes peeled and chopped into 1/4-inch cubes
2 garlic cloves, minced
1 bag spinach, washed
1/4 cup cream or milk
16 oz extra-firm tofu, crumbled
1/8 tsp turmeric
1/8 tsp salt
1/4 tsp freshly ground black pepper
1/4 tsp chili powder

Procedure

1 Add broth, potatoes and garlic to a medium pan. Cover pan. Bring to a boil and then simmer on low until potatoes are soft, about 15 minutes. Stir once every five minutes. Add spinach and sauté until spinach is wilted.

2 Preheat the oven to 375 degrees F while the potatoes and garlic are cooking.

3 Puree half the tofu with cream or milk, turmeric, salt, black pepper and chili powder in a food processor. Crumble the other half. Combine pureed tofu, remaining crumbled tofu, and spinach mixture in a 6x6-inch baking dish and mix thoroughly. Bake for 20 min. Remove from the oven and allow it to set for at least 10 min before serving.

Servings: 8
Yield: 8
Preparation Time: 10 minutes
Cooking Time: 20 minutes

Nutrition Facts

Serving size: 1/8 of a recipe (6.5 ounces).
Calories:113.92
Calories from fat:31.38
Carbs:13.92g
Protein: 8.62g

Creamy Fruit Smoothie

2 cups milk
1 1/2 cup fresh blue berries
1 large banana
2 Tbsp flax seeds
1 Tbsp agave nectar
Procedure
1 Combine all ingredients in a blender and blend until smooth and flaxseeds are ground.
Servings: 4
Yield: 4
Preparation Time: 5 minutes
Nutrition Facts
Serving size: 1/4 of a recipe (7.7 ounces).
Calories:154.23
Calories from fat:34.67
Carbs:26.69g
Protein:5.36g

Dinner

Sweet and Spicy Stir Fry with Chicken and Broccoli

Serve this dish-with-a-kick over brown jasmine rice.
3 cups broccoli florets
1 Tbsp olive oil
2 skinless, boneless chicken breast halves cut into 1 inch strips
1/4 cup sliced green onions
1 Tbsp hoisin sauce
1 Tbsp Chili paste 1 Tbsp Bragg's liquid aminos
1/2 tsp ground ginger

1/4 tsp crushed red pepper
1/2 tsp salt
1/2 tsp black pepper
1/8 cup chicken stock

Procedure

1 Place broccoli in a steamer over 1 inch of boiling water, and cover. Cook until tender but still firm, about 5 minutes.

2 Heat the oil in a skillet over medium heat, and sauté the chicken, green onions, and garlic until the chicken is no longer pink and juices run clear.

3 Stir the hoisin sauce, Chili paste, and Bragg's into the skillet. Add ginger, red pepper, salt, and black pepper. Stir in the chicken stock and simmer about 2 minutes. Mix in the steamed broccoli until coated with the sauce mixture.

Servings: 4
Yield: 4
Preparation Time: 10 minutes
Cooking Time: 20 minutes
Total Time: 30 minutes

Nutrition Facts

Serving size: 1/4 of a recipe (4.7 ounces).
Calories:139.61
Calories from fat:47.31
Carbs:7.58g
Protein: 15.94g

Baked Halibut

1 tsp olive oil
1 cup diced zucchini
1/2 cup minced onion
1 clove garlic peeled and minced
2 cups diced fresh tomatoes 2 Tbsp chopped fresh basil
1/4 tsp salt
1/4 tsp ground black pepper
4 (6 oz) halibut steaks
1/3 cup crumbled feta cheese

Procedure

1 Preheat oven to 450 degrees F (230 degrees C). Lightly grease a shallow baking dish.

2 Heat olive oil in a medium saucepan over medium heat and stir in zucchini, onion, and garlic. Cook and stir 5 minutes or until tender. Remove saucepan from heat and mix in tomatoes, basil, salt, and pepper.

3 Arrange halibut steaks in a single layer in the prepared baking dish. Spoon equal amounts of the zucchini mixture over each steak. Top with feta cheese.

4 Bake 15 minutes in the preheated oven, or until fish is easily flaked with a fork.

Servings: 4
Yield: 4
Preparation Time: 15 minutes
Cooking Time: 15 minutes
Total Time: 30 minutes

Nutrition Facts

Serving size: 1/4 of a recipe (12.6 ounces).
Calories:344.39
Calories from fat:141.09
Carbs:8.25g
Protein: 41.54g

Blackened Tuna Steaks

2 Tbsp olive oil
2 Tbsp lime juice
2 Cloves garlic minced
4 tuna steaks
1 fresh mango peeled, pitted and chopped
1/4 cup finely chopped red bell pepper
1/2 Spanish onion, finely chopped
1 green onion chopped
2 Tbsp chopped fresh cilantro
1 Jalapeno pepper seeded and minced
2 Tbsp lime juice 1 1/2 tsp olive oil
2 Tbsp paprika
1 Tbsp cayenne pepper
1 Tbsp onion powder
2 tsp salt
1 tsp ground black pepper
1 tsp dried thyme
1 tsp dried basil
1 tsp dried oregano
1 Tbsp garlic powder
4 Tbsp olive oil

Procedure

1 Whisk together the olive oil, lime juice, and garlic in a bowl. Rub the tuna steaks with the mixture. Place the steaks in a sealable container and chill in refrigerator 3 hours.

2 Combine the mango, bell pepper, Spanish onion, green onion, cilantro, and jalapeno pepper in a bowl; stir. Add the lime juice and 1 1/2 teaspoons olive oil and toss to combine. Chill in refrigerator 1 hour.

3 Stir together the paprika, cayenne pepper, onion powder, salt, pepper, thyme, basil, oregano, and garlic powder in a bowl. Remove the tuna steaks from the refrigerator and

gently rinse with water and then dip each side of each steak in the spice mixture to coat.

4 Heat 2 tablespoons olive oil in a large skillet over medium heat. Gently lay the tuna steaks into the hot oil. Cook the tuna on one side for 3 minutes; remove to a plate. Pour the remaining 2 tablespoons olive oil into the skillet and let it get hot. Lay the tuna with the uncooked side down into the skillet and cook another 3 minutes; remove from heat immediately.

5 Spoon about 1/2 cup of the mango salsa onto each of 4 plates. Lay the tuna steaks atop the salsa and serve immediately.

Servings: 4

Yield: 4

Preparation Time: 45 minutes

Cooking Time: 10 minutes

Total Time: 3 hours and 55 minutes

Nutrition Facts

Serving size: 1/4 of a recipe (5.4 ounces).

Calories:298.08

Calories from fat:212.04

Carbs:17.21g

Protein: 7.17g

Glazed Mahi Mahi

3 Tbsp agave nectar
3 Tbsp Bragg's liquid aminos
3 Tbsp balsamic vinegar
1 tsp grated fresh ginger root
1 clove garlic crushed or to taste 2 tsp olive oil
4 (6 oz) mahi mahi fillets
1 Tbsp vegetable oil salt and pepper to taste

Procedure

1 In a shallow glass dish, stir together the agave, Bragg's, balsamic vinegar, ginger, garlic and olive oil. Season fish fillets with salt and pepper, and place them into the dish. If the fillets have skin on them, place them skin side down. Cover, and refrigerate for 20 minutes to marinate.

2 Heat vegetable oil in a large skillet over medium-high heat. Remove fish from the dish, and reserve marinade. Fry fish for 4 to 6 minutes on each side, turning once, until fish flakes easily with a fork. Remove fillets to a serving platter and keep warm.

3 Pour reserved marinade into the skillet, and heat over medium heat until the mixture reduces to a glaze consistently. Spoon glaze over fish, and serve immediately.

Servings: 4
Yield: 4
Preparation Time: 5 minutes
Cooking Time: 12 minutes
Total Time: 37 minutes

Nutrition Facts

Serving size: 1/4 of a recipe (10.8 ounces).
Calories:355.43
Calories from fat:74.82
Carbs:16.38g
Protein: 50.98g

Grilled Salmon

1 1/2 pound salmon fillets
lemon pepper to taste
garlic powder to taste
salt to taste 1/3 cup Bragg's liquid aminos
1/3 cup agave nectar
1/3 cup water
1/4 cup olive oil
Procedure

1 Season salmon fillets with lemon pepper, garlic powder, and salt.

2 In a small bowl, stir together Bragg's, agave, water, and oil. Place fish in a large resealable plastic bag with the sauce mixture, seal, and turn to coat. Refrigerate for at least 2 hours.

3 Preheat grill for medium heat.

4 Lightly oil grill grate. Place salmon on the preheated grill, and discard marinade. Cook salmon for 6 to 8 minutes per side, or until the fish flakes easily with a fork.

Servings: 6
Yield: 6
Preparation Time: 15 minutes
Cooking Time: 16 minutes
Total Time: 2 hours
Nutrition Facts
Serving size: 1/6 of a recipe (5.7 ounces).
Calories:268.58
Calories from fat:124.60
Carbs:13.58g
Protein: 21.56g

Tuna Teriyaki

2 Tbsp Bragg's liquid aminos
1 Tbsp Chinese rice wine
1 large clove garlic minced
1 Tbsp minced fresh ginger root 4 (6 oz) tuna steaks (about 3/4 inch thick)
1 Tbsp olive oil

Procedure

1 In a shallow dish, stir together Bragg's, rice wine, garlic, and ginger. Place tuna in the marinade, and turn to coat. Cover, and refrigerate for at least 30 minutes.

2 Preheat grill for medium-high heat.

3 Remove tuna from marinade, and discard remaining liquid. Brush both sides of steaks with oil.

4 Cook tuna for approximately for 3 to 6 minutes per side, or to desired doneness.

Servings: 4
Yield: 4
Preparation Time: 15 minutes
Cooking Time: 12 minutes
Total Time: 57 minutes

Nutrition Facts

Serving size: 1/4 of a recipe (3.6 ounces).
Calories:163.67
Calories from fat:68.7
Carbs:1.91g
Protein:20.44g

Lemony Orange Roughy

A fast and simple recipe, yet a taste our whole family loves. Serve with a green salad.

1 Tbsp olive oil

4 (4 oz) fillets orange roughy

1 orange, juiced 1 lemon, juiced

1/2 tsp lemon pepper

Procedure

1 Heat oil in a large skillet over medium-high heat. Arrange fillets in the skillet, and drizzle with orange juice and lemon juice. Sprinkle with lemon pepper. Cook for 5 minutes, or until fish is easily flaked with a fork.

Servings: 4

Yield: 4

Preparation Time: 15 minutes

Cooking Time: 5 minutes

Total Time: 20 minutes

Nutrition Facts

Serving size: 1/4 of a recipe (4.4 ounces).

Calories:107.36

Calories from fat:35.84

Carbs:3.26g

Protein:15.14g

Baked Eggplant Salad

1 pound eggplant
2 red bell pepper
2 tomatoes seeded and chopped
2 cloves garlic, minced
1/4 cup finely chopped red onion
1/4 cup fresh parsley, finely chopped 2 tsp red wine vinegar
2 tsp Dijon mustard
1/2 tsp agave nectar
kosher or sea salt to taste black pepper to taste

Procedure

1 Preheat the oven to 400°F. Remove the stem from the eggplant and cut the eggplant in half and remove the seeds and membrane. Place the eggplant and peppers on a baking sheet covered with parchment paper and roast for about 25 to 30 min until soft. Place the peppers in a bowl and cover with plastic wrap, until cool enough to handle.

2 Peel the skin off the peppers and cut into strips. Scoop out the flesh of the eggplant and mash, and then drain any extra liquid.

3 Place the peppers and eggplant in a large bowl. Add the tomatoes, garlic, onion and parsley. In a small bowl, mix together the vinegar, mustard, agave, salt and black pepper. Pour the dressing onto the salad and mix well. Cover and refrigerate for at least 1 hour prior to serving.

Servings: 6
Preparation Time: 10 minutes plus 1hr resting time
Cooking Time: 50 minutes

Nutrition Facts

Serving size: 1/6 of a recipe (5.9 ounces).
Calories:45.58
Calories from fat:4.01
Carbs:9.7g
Protein:1.75g

Traffic Light Peppers

1 cup brown basmati rice
2 medium red bell pepper
2 medium yellow bell peppers
2 medium green bell peppers
1/4 cup vegetable broth
1 cup chopped onion
1 tsp chili powder
1 tsp ground cumin 1 tsp dried oregano
1/4 tsp sea salt
1/4 tsp ground black pepper
1 (15 oz) can black beans, drained and rinsed
1 cup brown rice, cooked
1 cup seeded and chopped tomato
8 slices Cheddar cheese

Procedure

1 Cook rice according to package directions.

2 Preheat the oven to 400°F.

3 Cut each bell pepper in half lengthwise. Remove seeds and ribs. Bring a large saucepan of water to a boil. Add the bell pepper halves and blanch for about 4 min. Drain and pat dry.

4 Heat the oil in a skillet over medium heat. Add the onion and sauté for about 3 min. Add chili powder, cumin, oregano, salt and black pepper. Sauté for 1 min. Add the beans, rice and tomato and sauté for 2 min.

5 Stuffed bell peppers with the mixture, packing them well. Top each bell pepper with a slice of cheese. Place in an 8x8-inch baking dish.

6 Bake bell peppers, uncovered for about 20 min. Set oven to a broil. Broil bell peppers for 1 to 2 min., until the top is browned and cheese is bubbly.

Servings: 4
Yield: 4
Preparation Time: 15 minutes

Cooking Time: 30 minutes

Nutrition Facts

Serving size: 1/4 of a recipe (17 ounces).

Calories:562.63

Calories from fat:190.41

Carbs:73.26g

Protein:24.63g

Stuffed Portobello Mushrooms with Brown Rice

1 cup short-grain brown rice
1/4 cup finely chopped onion
1/2 cup finely chopped carrot
1 tsp dried basil
1/2 tsp dried oregano
1/2 cup chopped red tomato
1/2 cup chopped yellow tomato 3 Tbsp finely chopped fresh parsley
1 Tbsp chopped fresh chives
1/2 tsp salt
½ tsp black pepper
4 Portobello mushrooms cap
Vegetable oil cooking spray
1/4 cup parmesan cheese

Procedure

1 Cook rice according to package directions. During the last 5 min. of cooking time, add onion, carrot, basil and oregano.

2 In a bowl, combine cooked rice, tomatoes, parsley, chives, salt and black pepper. Set aside. Preheat the oven broiler.

3 Remove the gills from the undersides of the mushrooms using a spoon; discard gills. Place the mushrooms, gill side down, on a foil lined broiler tray that has been coated with cooking spray. Broil mushrooms for about 5 min.

4 Turn mushrooms over and stuff each mushroom with equal amounts of the rice mixture. Sprinkle each with parmesan. Broil mushrooms for about 5 to 6 min. until lightly browned.

Servings: 4
Yield: 4
Preparation Time: 20 minutes
Cooking Time: 1 hour
Nutrition Facts
Serving size: 1/4 of a recipe (9.4 ounces).
Calories:222.72
Calories from fat:27.93
Carbs:46.88g
Protein:6.33g

Spinach, Beet and Orange Salad

For the Dressing:
4 Tbsp rice vinegar
2 Tbsp agave nectar
2 tsp paprika
2 tsp fresh ginger, grated
1/2 tsp chili powder 1 lime, juiced
For the Salad:
1/2 can beets (plain, unpickled)
6 cups baby spinach
2 mandarin oranges
Procedure

1 Whisk the vinegar, agave nectar, paprika, ginger, and chili powder in a saucepan and bring to a boil. Add lime juice. Let dressing cool.

2 Arrange spinach on a platter and top with beets and oranges. Drizzle dressing over the spinach salad.

Servings: 4
Preparation Time: 20 minutes
Cooking Time: 1 hour and 20 minutes

Nutrition Facts
Serving size: 1/4 of a recipe (16.3 ounces).
Calories:205.33
Calories from fat:37.36
Carbs:44.03g
Protein:10.41g

Strawberry and Feta Salad

1 cup slivered almonds
2 cloves garlic -- minced
1 tsp Dijon mustard
1/4 cup raspberry vinegar
2 Tbsp balsamic vinegar
2 Tbsp agave nectar
1/2 cup olive oil
1 head romaine lettuce, torn
1 pint fresh strawberries, sliced
1 cup crumbled feta cheese
Procedure
1 In a skillet over medium-high heat, cook the almonds, stirring frequently, until lightly toasted. Remove from heat, and set aside.
2 Place the garlic, Dijon mustard, raspberry vinegar, balsamic vinegar, agave and olive oil in a blender and blend for 15 seconds.
3 In a large bowl, toss together the toasted almonds, romaine lettuce, strawberries, and feta cheese. Cover with the dressing mixture, and toss to serve.
Servings: 10
Preparation Time: 15 minutes
Total Time: 15 minutes
Nutrition Facts
Serving size: 1/10 of a recipe (6.9 ounces).
Calories:270.18
Calories from fat:187.95

Carbs:15.69g
Protein:6.43g

Dessert

Chocolate Cherry Dessert

1 cup frozen cherries
1 banana
3/4 cup milk
Procedure
1 Put all ingredients into a blender and blend until smooth.
Servings: 4
Preparation Time: 5 minutes
Nutrition Facts
Serving size: 1/4 of a recipe (4 ounces).
Calories:66.96
Calories from fat:10.35
Carbs:13.2g
Protein:2.19g

Fresh Blueberry Pie

11/3 cup pitted dates
1 1/2 Tbsp orange juice
2 cups graham cracker crumbs, coarsely crushed
2 Tbsp agave nectar
3 1/2 cup blueberries
1/4 tsp ground cinnamon 2 cups strawberries, sliced
Banana Cashew Cream
1/4 banana
1/4 cup raw cashews, soaked for at least 6 hours

Procedure

1 Puree the dates and orange juice in a food processor or blender.

2 Mash the date puree and graham cracker crumbs together with your hands to combine. Pat the crust into a glass pie dish.

3 Stir together the agave nectar, berries and cinnamon. Add the remaining date puree, and sliced strawberries. Spread the mixture in the pie dish and refrigerate for 2 hours.

4 Top each slice with a dollop of Banana Cashew Cream.

5 To make the Banana Cashew Cream: Blend the banana and cashews with 2 tbsp water in a food processor or blender until creamy. Refrigerate until ready to use.

Servings: 8

Preparation Time: 2 hours and 20 minutes

Nutrition Facts

Serving size: 1/8 of a recipe (3.5 ounces).

Calories:136.36

Calories from fat:42.16

Carbs:23.41g

Protein:2.34g

Snacks

Tomatillo and Cilantro Salsa

This makes a wonderful dip. Serve with warm queso cheese and tortilla chips. Make sure to overload with the cheese to ensure a good protein balance.

1 small red onion chopped

1 1/2 pound fresh tomatillos, husks removed, chopped

2 jalapeño pepper, stems and seeds removed, chopped 1 cup packed cilantro leaves and tender stems

1 lime, juiced

1 tsp salt

Procedure

1 Process all ingredients in a food processor until smooth.

Yield: 4 1/2 cups

Preparation Time: 5 minutes

Nutrition Facts

Serving size: Entire recipe (39 ounces).

Calories:346.65

Calories from fat:63.38

Carbs:69.84g

Protein:10.34g

Guacamole

3 avocados peeled, pitted and mashed
1 lime juice
1 tsp salt
1/2 cup diced red onion 3 Tbsp chopped fresh cilantro
2 roma (plum) tomatoes, diced
1 tsp minced garlic
1 pinch ground cayenne pepper

Procedure

1 In a medium bowl, mash together the avocados, lime juice, and salt. Mix in onion, cilantro, tomatoes, and garlic. Stir in cayenne pepper. Refrigerate 1 hour for best flavor, or serve immediately.

Servings: 4
Yield: 4
Preparation Time: 10 minutes
Total Time: 10 minutes

Nutrition Facts

Serving size: 1/4 of a recipe (8.7 ounces).
Calories:263.74
Calories from fat:186.27
Carbs:17.98g
Protein:3.92g

Peach Smoothie

2 cups milk
1 cup chopped fresh peaches
1/4 tsp almond extract 2 Tbsp flax seeds
1 Tbsp agave nectar
Procedure
1 Combine all ingredients in a blender and blend until smooth and the flax seeds are ground.
Servings: 4
Preparation Time: 5 minutes
Nutrition Facts
Serving size: 1/4 of a recipe (6.2 ounces).
Calories:125.97
Calories from fat:46.86
Carbs:15.97g
Protein:5.53g

Pico De Gallo

1 large sweet onion , chopped
15 (about 2 pounds) roma (plum) tomatoes, chopped
2 jalapeño peppers, seeded and chopped 1 cup cilantro, chopped
1 tsp salt
2 Tbsp lemon juice
Procedure
1 Mix all ingredients together in a large bowl and serve.
Servings: 7
Yield: 7
Preparation Time: 20 minutes
Nutrition Facts
Serving size: 1/7 of a recipe (15.8 ounces).
Calories:88.28
Calories from fat:7.32

Carbs:19.42g
Protein:3.96g

Soup

Mulligatawny

1/2 cup chopped onion
2 stalks celery chopped
1 carrot diced
1/4 cup butter
1 1/2 Tbsp all purpose flour
1 1/2 tsp curry powder
4 cups organic chicken broth 1/2 apple cored and chopped
1/4 cup white rice uncooked
1 skinless, boneless organic chicken breast half cut into cubes
salt to taste
ground black pepper to taste
1 pinch dried thyme
1/2 cup heavy cream, heated

Procedure

1 Sauté onions, celery, carrot, and butter in a large soup pot. Add flour and curry, and cook 5 more minutes. Add chicken broth, mix well, and bring to a boil. Simmer 30 minutes.

2 Add apple, rice, chicken, salt, pepper, and thyme. Simmer 15-20 minutes, or until rice is done. Remove from heat.

3 Add hot cream and stir.

Servings: 6
Yield: 6
Preparation Time: 20 minutes

Cooking Time: 1 hour
Total Time: 1 hour
Nutrition Facts
Serving size: 1/6 of a recipe (9.4 ounces).
Calories:242.02
Calories from fat:147.29
Carbs:13.79g
Protein:9.4g

Pasta Fagioli

3 Tbsp olive oil
1 onion quartered and halved
2 cloves garlic minced
1 (29 oz) can tomato sauce
5 1/2 cup water
1 Tbsp dried parsley
1 1/2 tsp dried basil 1 1/2 tsp dried oregano
1 tsp salt
1 (15 oz) can cannellini beans
1 (15 oz) can navy beans
1/3 cup grated Parmesan cheese
1/2 pound ditalini pasta, wholegrain
Procedure

1 In a large pot over medium heat, cook onion in olive oil until translucent. Stir in garlic and cook until tender. Reduce heat, and stir in tomato sauce, water, parsley, basil, oregano, salt, cannellini beans, navy beans and Parmesan. Simmer 1 hour.

2 Bring a large pot of lightly salted water to a boil. Add pasta and cook for 8 to 10 minutes or until al dente; drain. Stir into soup.

Servings: 8
Yield: 8
Preparation Time: 10 minutes
Cooking Time: 1 hour and 30 minutes

Total Time: 1 hour and 40 minutes
Nutrition Facts
Serving size: 1/8 of a recipe (11.6 ounces).
Calories:250.5
Calories from fat:61.19
Carbs:34.85g
Protein:14.02g

Cream of Tomato Basil Soup

4 tomatoes peeled, seeded and diced
4 cups tomato juice
14 leaves fresh basil
1/2 cup milk 1/2 cup heavy whipping cream
1/2 cup butter
salt and pepper to taste
Procedure

1 Place tomatoes and juice in a stock pot over medium heat. Simmer for 30 minutes. Puree the tomato mixture along with the basil leaves, and return the puree to the stock pot.

2 Place the pot over medium heat, and stir in the milk, heavy cream and butter. Season with salt and pepper. Heat, stirring until the butter is melted. Do not boil.

Servings: 4
Yield: 4
Preparation Time: 10 minutes
Cooking Time: 35 minutes
Total Time: 45 minutes
Nutrition Facts
Serving size: 1/4 of a recipe (17.7 ounces).
Calories:428.41
Calories from fat:313.54
Carbs:26.51g
Protein:8.68g

Slow-Cooker Chicken Tortilla Soup

1 pound shredded cooked organic chicken
1 (15 oz) can Rotel diced tomatoes with habanero
1 (10 oz) can enchilada sauce
1 medium onion chopped
1 (4 ounce) can chopped green chili peppers
2 cloves garlic minced
2 cups water
1 (14.5 oz) can organic chicken broth
2 tsp cumin
1 tsp chili powder 1 tsp salt
1/4 tsp black pepper
1 bay leaf
1 (10 oz) package frozen corn
1 can (15 oz) black beans
1 Tbsp chopped cilantro
7 corn tortillas
vegetable oil
1 cup cheese, grated Mexican
1 avocado diced

Procedure

1 Place chicken, tomatoes, enchilada sauce, onion, green chilies, and garlic into a slow cooker. Pour in water and chicken broth, and season with cumin, chili powder, salt, pepper, and bay leaf. Stir in corn and cilantro. Cover, and cook on Low setting for 6 to 8 hours or on High setting for 3 to 4 hours.

2 Preheat oven to 400 degrees F (200 degrees C).

3 Lightly brush both sides of tortillas with oil. Cut tortillas into strips, and then spread on a baking sheet.

4 Bake in preheated oven until crisp, about 10 to 15 minutes. To serve, sprinkle cheese, tortilla strips and avocado over soup.

Servings: 8

Preparation Time: 30 minutes

Cooking Time: 8 hours
Total Time: 8 hours and 30 minutes
Nutrition Facts
Serving size: 1/8 of a recipe (12.3 ounces).
Calories:306.15
Calories from fat:96.14
Carbs:26.7g
Protein:26.7g

Southwest Soup

1 cup mixed vegetables [peppers, onions, carrots etc]
1 can (15 oz) chopped tomatoes
1 can (15 oz) black beans
2 cups water
1 tsp vegetable bouillon
1/8 tsp black pepper
1/8 tsp cayenne pepper 1 Tbsp chili powder
1/4 tsp garlic powder
1/4 tsp salt
1/4 tsp oregano
1 pinch cumin seeds
2 chicken breasts, chopped
Procedure
1 Combine ingredients in a slow cooker and cook for 4 hours on "High."
Servings: 8
Yield: 8
Nutrition Facts
Serving size: 1/8 of a recipe (10.5 ounces).
Calories:153.62
Calories from fat:19.78
Carbs:17.55g
Protein:17.31g

Squash Bisque

4 1/2 cup winter squash, peeled, seeded and cubed into ¼" chunks

1 cup chopped onion

3 1/4 cup vegetable broth

2 cloves garlic, minced

1 tsp ground cardamom 1 1/2 tsp ground cumin

1/4 tsp ground nutmeg

1/4 tsp cayenne pepper or to taste

1 tsp salt

1/4 cup sour cream

Procedure

1 Preheat the oven to 375°F.

2 Place squash in a baking dish and bake for 30 min. or until tender. Set aside.

3 In a large stock pot, sauté the onion 1/4 cup broth over medium heat until translucent, about 3 min. Add garlic, cardamom, cumin, nutmeg, cayenne and salt. Sauté for 2 to 3 min. Put in the cooked squash. Add the remaining 3 cups broth.

4 Puree the soup in batches in a food processor or blender until smooth.

5 Return soup to pot and bring to a boil. Turn down to simmer, partially cover pot, and simmer for 10 min or until heated thoroughly.

6 Garnish the top of each bowl of soup with 1 tbsp sour cream.

Servings: 6

Yield: 6

Preparation Time: 30 minutes

Cooking Time: 50 minutes

Nutrition Facts

Serving size: 1/6 of a recipe (10.3 ounces).

Calories:96.22

Calories from fat:6.14

Carbs:21.71g
Protein:2.93g

Spicy Chicken Soup

2 quarts water
8 skinless, boneless organic chicken breast halves
1/2 tsp salt
1 tsp ground black pepper
1 tsp garlic powder
2 Tbsp dried parsley
1 Tbsp onion powder
5 cubes chicken bouillon
3 Tbsp olive oil
1 onion chopped 3 cloves garlic chopped
1 (16 oz) jar chunky salsa
2 (14.5 oz) can peeled and diced tomatoes
1 (14.5 oz) can whole peeled tomatoes
1 (10.75 oz) can diced tomatoes
3 Tbsp chili powder
1 (15 oz) can whole kernel corn drained
2 (16 oz) can chili beans, undrained
1 (8 oz) container sour cream

Procedure

1 In a large pot over medium heat, combine water, chicken, salt, pepper, garlic powder, parsley, onion powder and bouillon cubes. Bring to a boil, then reduce heat and simmer 1 hour, or until chicken juices run clear. Remove chicken, reserve broth. Shred chicken.

2 In a large pot over medium heat, cook onion and garlic in olive oil until slightly browned. Stir in salsa, diced tomatoes, whole tomatoes, tomatoes, chili powder, corn, chili beans, sour cream, shredded chicken and 5 cups broth. Simmer 30 minutes.

Servings: 8
Yield: 8

Preparation Time: 15 minutes
Cooking Time: 30 minutes
Total Time: 45 minutes
Nutrition Facts
Serving size: 1/8 of a recipe (28.6 ounces).
Calories:565.02
Calories from fat:216.16
Carbs:28.3g
Protein:58.64g

Vegetable, Fruit and Lentil Soup

1/4 cup butter
2 large sweet potatoes peeled and chopped into ¼ inch cubes
3 large carrot peeled and chopped
1 apple peeled, cored and chopped
1 onion chopped
1/2 cup red lentils
1/2 tsp minced fresh ginger 1/2 tsp ground black pepper
1 tsp salt
1/2 tsp ground cumin
1/2 tsp chili powder
1/2 tsp paprika
4 cups vegetable broth
plain yogurt
Procedure

1 Melt the butter in a large, heavy bottomed pot over medium-high heat. Place the chopped sweet potatoes, carrots, apple, and onion in the pot. Stir and cook the apples and vegetables until the onions are translucent, about 10 minutes.

2 Stir the lentils, ginger, ground black pepper, salt, cumin, chili powder, paprika, and vegetable broth into the pot with the apple and vegetable mixture. Bring the soup to a boil over high heat, and then reduce the heat to medium-low,

cover, and simmer until the lentils and vegetables are soft, about 30 minutes.

3 Puree the soup with a hand blender.

4 Continue simmering over medium-high heat, about 10 minutes. Add water as needed to thin the soup to your preferred consistency. Serve with yogurt for garnish.

Servings: 6

Yield: 6

Preparation Time: 20 minutes

Cooking Time: 50 minutes

Total Time: 1 hour and 10 minutes

Nutrition Facts

Serving size: 1/6 of a recipe (12.3 ounces).

Calories:284.94

Calories from fat:98.44

Carbs:39.95g

Protein:8.22g

Vegetarian Tortilla Soup

2 Tbsp vegetable oil
1 pound package frozen pepper and onion stir fry mix
2 garlic clove, minced
3 Tbsp ground cumin
1 can crushed tomatoes with chili peppers
3 cans chopped green chili peppers, drained
4 cans vegetable broth ½ tsp ea. Salt and pepper
1 can whole kernel corn
12 ounces tortilla chips
1 cup shredded Cheddar cheese
1 avocado peeled, pitted and diced

Procedure

1 Heat the oil in a large pot over medium heat. Stir in the pepper and onion stir fry mix, garlic, and cumin, and cook 5 minutes, until vegetables are tender. Mix in the tomatoes and chili peppers. Pour in the broth, and salt and pepper. Bring to a boil, reduce heat to low, and simmer 30 minutes.

Servings: 12
Yield: 12
Preparation Time: 15 minutes
Cooking Time: 40 minutes
Total Time: 55 minutes

Nutrition Facts

Serving size: 1/12 of a recipe (2 ounces). Calories:315
Calories from fat:139.43
Carbs:37.2g
Protein:8.7g

Preparing for your appointment

Although Gilbert's Syndrome is not a severe disorder, it is important that you talk with experts to help you deal with its symptoms. This will help you understand that your genetic disorder is common and there's no need for you to stress yourself in worrying for complications.

If a recent series of blood examinations revealed that you may be positive of Gilbert's syndrome, you should prepare yourself in meeting your doctor. To acquire the necessary information that you need, list down problems and inquiries that you can talk to your doctor about. Here are suggested questions that you can ask your doctor and can help facilitate a discussion:

a. What is your bilirubin level? Is your bilirubin level significantly increased?

b. Should you undergo another bilirubin level test?

c. You've been experiencing some unexplained symptoms, could these be triggered by Gilbert's syndrome?

d. Is your medication compatible for Gilbert's syndrome? Do these drugs expose you to increased risk of complications?

e. Do you need treatment for Gilbert's syndrome? Is there a cure for this disorder?

f. Can Gilbert's syndrome cause complications or lead to liver damage? What are possible diseases that are associated with this syndrome?

g. Is there anything that you can do to maintain a low bilirubin level?

h. What are signs and symptoms can you expect if your bilirubin levels increase?

i. If obvious symptoms appear such as jaundice, should you make an appointment with the doctor?

j. What is the likelihood that your children or other relatives also acquire Gilbert's syndrome?

Where can you get information?

Your healthcare provider can give you the best information that you need. Sources of information for questions and concerns related this medical problem is available. Many websites offer educational materials for patients and professional levels. Under the patient level, you will be provided with the basics and general overview of the disorder as well as longer, more detailed and sophisticated discussions about your condition. These materials work best if you want in-depth information. On the other hand, many websites also offer further information and continuing education to keep doctors and other health professionals updated with the latest medical findings. With thorough, long and complex articles containing multiple references, your doctor can be more effective in helping you with your disorder.

In addition, you can refer to the following books recommended to help you:

- *"The Liver Cleansing Diet"*. It contains eight week eating plan to improve liver function and care for your liver cells.
- *"The Healthy Liver and Bowel Book"*. This book actually offers liver friendly recipes for healthier diet and vital principles that you can follow in long term for a healthy liver. More detailed information is also available to explain specific conditions.
- *"Raw Juices Can Save Your Life"*. This juice book contains carefully designed juices to help you with common health problems. Also, this highlights a complete A to Z guide of diseases and their specific healing juices.

As you deal with the symptoms of Gilbert's syndrome, you should acquire proper awareness and seek professional help. To avoid complications, inform your doctor regarding your condition. You should also keep in mind that this disorder is still considered falling within the normal range of variations in the body. Since this is genetically acquired, you cannot avoid the occurrence but you can definitely manage the symptoms. Living a healthy lifestyle will greatly help you combat Gilbert's syndrome. Coordinate with your doctor, help yourself and continue to uphold good health for longer and better life with your family and loved ones around you.

Internet Resources / Further Reading

The following Internet resources may be helpful in answering any health or medical questions you may have. The sites were chosen because of their superior content, accuracy, and authority.

Print Publications Online

American Family Physician

http://www.aafp.org/online/en/home/publications/journals/afp.html

A full-text, online version of the esteemed journal. Contains excellent review articles on clinical medicine. Many come with patient education information.

Merck Manual of Diagnosis and Therapy, 17th ed.

http://www.merck.com/mmpe/index.html

A medical guide for professionals, available online. Contains technical information for a host of diseases along with their corresponding diagnosis and treatment suggestions.

Merck Manual of Geriatrics

http://www.merck.com/mkgr/mmg/home.jsp

Similar in format to the Merck Manual of Diagnosis and Therapy, this guide focuses on disorders and diseases with a slant towards implications for the elderly.

Merck Manual of Medical Information - 2nd Home Edition

http://www.merck.com/mmhe/index.html

A consumers' guide to diseases and their treatments. This is a complete online version of the text edition, with videos and a pronunciation guide

Postgraduate Medicine

http://www.postgradmed.com/

Professional medical journal with review articles on diseases and treatments. Although this is directed to the professional, the journal includes patient notes which are directed toward the general consumer.

MEDLINE/MedlinePlus

http://www.nlm.nih.gov/medlineplus/

Anatomy videos aimed at the general consumer plus thousands of articles on a variety of health related topics.

PubMed

http://www.ncbi.nlm.nih.gov/sites/entrez

PubMed comprises more than 20 million citations for biomedical literature from MEDLINE, life science journals, and online books. Citations may include links to full-text content from PubMed Central and publisher web sites.

News Services

These sources offer reliable information and up to date news stories about medical research.

Understanding Medical News

Consumer's Guide to Taking Charge of Medical Information

http://www.health-insight-harvard.org/

This guide, developed by the Harvard School of Public Health, helps you to decipher "scary" headlines.

Deciphering Medspeak

http://mlanet.org/resources/medspeak/index.html

To make informed health decisions, you have probably read a newspaper or magazine article, tuned into a radio or television program, or searched the Internet to find answers to health questions. If so, you have probably encountered "medspeak," the specialized language of health professionals. The Medical Library Association developed "Deciphering Medspeak" to help translate common "medspeak" terms.

HealthNewsReviews

http://www.healthnewsreview.org/

HealthNewsReview.org is a website dedicated to:

- Improving the accuracy of news stories about medical treatments, tests, products and procedures.

- Helping consumers evaluate the evidence for and against new ideas in health care.

Interpreting News on Diet and Nutrition

http://www.hsph.harvard.edu/nutritionsource/nutrition-news/media/

Confused by all the conflicting stories about what's good to eat and what's not? Sensational headlines don't always tell the whole story. Look at how nutrition news fits into the bigger scientific picture.

. *Understanding Risk. What Do Those Headlines Really Mean?*

http://www.niapublications.org/tipsheets/pdf/Understanding_Risk-What_Do_Those_Headlines_Really_Mean.pdf

Tipsheet that discusses the differences among types of clinical research and explains the significance of types of risk in research results. Excellent easy to understand information about risk.

Beyond the Headlines: What Consumers Need To Know About Nutrition News

http://www.foodinsight.org/

The International Food Information Council Foundation is dedicated to the mission of effectively communicating science-based information on health, food safety and nutrition for the public good.

Recommended Online News Sources

Aetna InteliHealth Health News

http://www.intelihealth.com/IH/ihtIH/WSIHW000/333/333.html?k=menux408x333

Top news headlines for the day. There is a section with commentaries written by Harvard Medical School physicians of several of the day's top news stories.

CNN Health

http://www.cnn.com/HEALTH/

Daily updated articles from a variety of news sources with links to related CNN stories and websites.

1st Headlines - Top Health Headlines

http://www.1stheadlines.com/health.htm

Top news stories from a variety of sources. Story may be covered by more than one news sources, allowing you to compare stories and fill in information gaps.

Reuters Health eLine

http://www.reutershealth.com/en/index.html

Daily medical news for the consumer (free) and for the professional (requires a subscription fee).

News Sources with Daily or Weekly Email Delivery

MedlinePlus Health News

http://www.nlm.nih.gov/medlineplus/

Produced by the National Library of Medicine, this site has daily news releases from sources such as United Press International, New York Times Syndicate, and Reuters. Stories can be retrieved for thirty days from publication.

Users may sign up for daily email of "Health Headlines" in several different categories.

Medscape

http://www.medscape.com/

From WebMD, a website for doctors with a comprehensive news feature. Go to the website to read the daily news or sign up for any of the forty free newsletters for delivery to your email address. There are newsletters in twenty-five specialties, a weekly multi-specialty edition, health business news, and much more.

NewsWise

http://feeds.feedburner.com/NewswiseMednews
Medical news stories. Information from news releases of more than four hundred universities, professional associations, and research institutions. Register and sign up to receive weekly medical news digests via email.

Alternative Medicine Ask Dr. Weil

http://www.drweil.com/

The popular doctor discusses alternative healing remedies for many common ailments.

Alternative Medicine Homepage

http://www.pitt.edu/~cbw/altm.html
From the Falk Library of the Health Sciences, University of Pittsburgh - a jumpstation for sources of information on unconventional, alternative, complementary, innovative, and integrative therapies.

HerbMed

http://www.herbmed.org/

HerbMed is an interactive, electronic herbal database. It provides hyperlinked access to the scientific & medical research articles on the use of herbs for treating medical conditions. This evidence-based information resource is for professionals, researchers, and the general public.

National Center for Complementary and Alternative Medicine

http://nccam.nih.gov/

General information about alternative and complementary therapies with links to research studies currently being conducted on alternative therapies for a variety of conditions.

Rosenthal Center for Complementary and Alternative Medicine

http://www.rosenthal.hs.columbia.edu//

Links to resources on acupuncture, homeopathy, chiropractic, and herbal medicine and alternative therapies for cancer and women's health. The Center sponsors research on alternative and complementary medical practices.

Clinical Research Trials

Center Watch

http://www.centerwatch.com/

Information on over 41,000 clinical trials for twenty disease categories. Profiles of 150 research centers conducting clinical trials and profiles of companies that provide a variety of contract services to the clinical trials industry. Includes industry and government sponsored clinical trials and information on new drug treatments approved by the Food and Drug Administration.

Clinical Trials

http://www.clinicaltrials.gov/

Information on current research being conducted on treatments for different diseases. Browse by disease category and sponsor or search the entire site. Learn what clinical trials are all about and how to decide to participate in a trial.

Diseases, Medical Conditions, General Health

Aetna Intelihealth

http://www.intellihealth.com/IH/ihtIH?t=408

From the Harvard Medical School, information on diseases and medical conditions, health and fitness, medications, nutrition, childbirth, and other topics.

Healthfinder

http://www.healthfinder.gov/

From the U.S. Department of Health and Human Services, a gateway to consumer information on diseases, medical conditions, health promotion, and many other topics.

Mayo Clinic

http://www.mayoclinic.com/

From the famed Mayo Clinic, information on diseases and conditions, treatment decisions, drugs and supplements, healthy living, and health assessment tools. Special features include online videos of exercises, diagnostic tests, surgical procedures, and medical conditions, healthy recipes, and self-care information.

National Organization for Rare Diseases

http://www.rarediseases.org/

Basic information on rare diseases and disorders. Full-reports are available for a fee.

NOAH (New York Online Access to Health)

http://www.noah-health.org/

English and Spanish language information and resources from organizations and governmental agencies. Aging, cancer, asthma, eye diseases, foot and ankle disorders, and pain are just a few of the topics covered.

Health Care Providers

American Board of Medical Specialties (ABMS)

http://www.abms.org/

Verify the certification status of any physician in the 24 specialities of the ABMS. Registration is required (free) and user is limited to five searches in a 24 hour period.

AMA Physician Select

https://extapps.ama-assn.org/doctorfinder/recaptcha.jsp

Gives credentials of MD's and DO's including medical school, year of graduation, and specialties.

American Hospital Directory

http://www.ahd.com/

Profiles of U.S. hospitals. Basic service is free; more detailed information by paid subscription only.

Federation of State Medical Boards

http://www.fsmb.org/

Select "Public Services" from the left-hand index, then select "Directory of State Medical Boards" to find links to web sites for the 50 U.S. States, plus the District of Columbia, Guam, and the Northern Mariana Islands. Not all of the states have physician profile or disciplinary action information. There are also links to osteopathic physician sites when available.

Health Pages

http://www.healthpages.com/

Information about physicians, dentists, hospitals and clinics, elder care facilities, dietitians and nutritionists.

Joint Commission on the Accreditation of Healthcare Organizations

http://www.jointcommission.org/

The Quality Check feature on this site supplies details on individual hospital performance ratings from JCAHO's accreditation reports. View Performance Reports and compare institutions' ratings. Reports cover hospitals, nursing homes, ambulatory care facilities, home care, laboratory services, and long term care facilities.

Nursing Home Compare

http://www.medicare.gov/NHCompare/Include/DataSection/Questions/SearchCriteriaNEW.asp?version=default&browser=Chrome|6|WinNT&language=English&defaultstatus=0&pagelist=Home&CookiesEnabledStatus=True
Provides detailed information about the performance of every Medicare and Medicaid certified nursing home in the country. Searchable by state. Includes a guide to choosing a nursing home and a nursing home checklist to help in making informed choices.

Questions and Answers about Health Insurance: A Consumer Guide

http://www.ahrq.gov/consumer/insuranceqa/

Questions and answers on choosing and using a health plan.

Quackery and Health Fraud

Quackwatch

http://www.quackwatch.com/

Want information about whether those alternative therapies work? This site has information on health fraud, medical quackery, "new age" medicine and "alternative" and "complementary" medicine.

National Council against Health Fraud

http://www.ncahf.org/

Non-profit voluntary health agency focusing on health fraud, misinformation, and quackery as public health oncerns. Read their position papers on acupuncture, homepathy, chiropractic, and other health issues.

Surgery

American College of Surgeons

http://www.facs.org/

Public information section offers guidelines on choosing a qualified surgeon.

Tests and Procedures - MedlinePlus

http://www.nlm.nih.gov/medlineplus/tutorial.html_

_ Interactive tutorials on 24 common tests and diagnostic procedures and more than 30 surgeries and treatment procedures.

CPSIA information can be obtained
at www.ICGtesting.com
Printed in the USA
BVHW041948271219
567993BV00013B/518/P